BREATHING FOR PEAK PERFORMANCE

Functional Exercises for Dance, Yoga, and Pilates

Eric Franklin

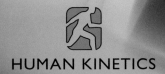

HUMAN KINETICS

Library of Congress Cataloging-in-Publication Data

Names: Franklin, Eric N., author.

Title: Breathing for peak performance : functional exercises for dance, yoga, and pilates / Eric Franklin.

Description: Champaign, IL : Human Kinetics, 2019.

Identifiers: LCCN 2018028443 (print) | LCCN 2018035443 (ebook) | ISBN 9781492569688 (e-book) | ISBN 9781492569671 (print)

Subjects: LCSH: Breathing exercises. | Dance. | Hatha yoga. | Pilates method.

Classification: LCC RA782 (ebook) | LCC RA782 .F7299 2019 (print) | DDC 613/.192--dc23

LC record available at https://lccn.loc.gov/2018028443

ISBN: 978-1-4925-6967-1 (print)

Acquisitions Editor: Bethany J. Bentley; **Managing Editor:** Kirsten E. Keller; **Copyeditor:** Joanna Hatzopoulos Portman; **Graphic Designer:** Joe Buck; **Cover Designer:** Keri Evans; **Cover Design Associate:** Susan Rothermel Allen; **Photograph (cover):** Kyle Monk/Blend Images/Getty Images; **Photographs (interior):** © Mindy Tucker; **Photo model:** Laura Hames Franklin; **Photo Asset Manager:** Laura Fitch; **Photo Production Manager:** Jason Allen; **Senior Art Manager:** Kelly Hendren; **Illustrations:** Sonja Burger, Joanna Culley, © Franklin Method; **Printer:** Premier Print Group

Human Kinetics books are available at special discounts for bulk purchase. Special editions or book excerpts can also be created to specification. For details, contact the Special Sales Manager at Human Kinetics.

Printed in the United States of America

10 9 8 7 6 5 4 3 2 1

Human Kinetics

P.O. Box 5076
Champaign, IL 61825-5076
Website: www.HumanKinetics.com

In the United States, email info@hkusa.com or call 800-747-4457.
In Canada, email info@hkcanada.com.
In the United Kingdom/Europe, email hk@hkeurope.com.

For information about Human Kinetics' coverage in other areas of the world, please visit our website: **www.HumanKinetics.com**

E7356

Contents

Introduction

Breathing is essential to your survival. Without food you can survive for several weeks; without water you can survive for three days; but without breathing you can survive only a few minutes. Nevertheless, when it comes to personal health, people tend to focus on nutrition and exercise while learning how to breathe more effectively receives little attention.

Breathing is necessary for energy production, which takes place in the cells of your body. Breathing also helps with functions that you may not think about. For example, breathing is necessary for speech production and for modulating abdominal pressure, which is important for movement and stability of the body and essential during birthing. When you do not breathe well, your health is compromised.

People take about 20,000 breaths a day. Therefore, improving your breathing brings noticeable benefits to every aspect of your daily life. Generally better breathing makes your life more comfortable. It makes you more alert and energetic, and it improves exercise and sport performance.

Understanding Healthy Breathing

Humans are naturally built for healthy breathing. The body evolved to breathe well before people created exercise systems for it. Therefore, all breathing cues are opinions on how to breathe well; they can help or they can hinder breathing performance. To cue breathing effectively, you must truly understand these cues rather than adopt them without scrutiny.

The ideas and exercises in this book are tried and tested over 30 years of teaching. A diverse population has used them, including dancers, yoga practitioners, Pilates instructors, actors, vocal coaches, physical therapists, athletes, horseback riders, tai chi practitioners, and midwives. In order to improve your breathing or coach someone who needs to improve, you need a solid understanding of anatomy, starting with the functional anatomy of breathing.

Healthy breathing is flexible and adaptive and can provide the human organism with sufficient energy under constantly changing conditions. Imagine running to catch a bus. Your breathing has very little time to adapt while your metabolism ramps up rapidly. If all the muscles and joints involved in breathing are sufficiently flexible and responsive, it is no problem. However, if you are stressed, tense, have bad posture, do not move enough, have a breathing disorder, or received instruction that impedes your breathing, it can be a challenge.

To improve breathing, you must first recognize and then remove the habits that hinder efficient breathing. To begin, explore the following behaviors that can make breathing less effective. They are best performed in a standing position.

- *Tension:* Notice your breathing. Proceed to clench your fists and curl your toes. Notice how your breathing becomes shallow. As soon as you relax, your breathing becomes easier. Grip your shoulders, and notice the effect on your breathing. Your goal is to reduce tension in your body that is impeding your breathing.

- *Poor Posture:* Notice your breathing. Slouch your shoulders, and notice how this posture affects your breathing. Shift your pelvis forward, and lean back with your upper body. Notice that it is harder to breathe under these circumstances. Good breathing requires good posture.

- *Negative Thinking:* Notice your breathing. Think, "I feel stressed!" Notice how your breath responds. Think, "I feel calm and relaxed." Notice how your breath responds to these contrasting messages. You are going to learn to use your thinking to support good breathing.

The Evolution of Breathing

The first water-living animals breathed through their skin. This method worked fine if they were small enough and plenty of flowing water was available. Some early animals that lived in fresh water started to move around a lot, so breathing through the skin was not sufficient. Multiple folded flaps (gills) developed to increase the surface area for absorption of oxygen. These gills were enhanced by primitive expansions of the pharynx (the part of the throat behind the nose and mouth) into early lungs. However, gills are not suited for breathing in air, and primitive air-breathing animals such as frogs had to rely on swallowing movements to gulp in air (figure I.1).

The breakthrough came with the advent of negative-pressure breathing, called thoracic breathing. The ribs attached themselves to the sternum in front, creating an expandable rib cage. This adaptation allowed the ribs to rotate and swivel toward the head for inhalation and reverse this action for exhalation. This movement, which is like lifting a bucket handle, increased the side-to-side diameter of the rib cage, creating a vacuum in the lungs and causing the air to rush in.

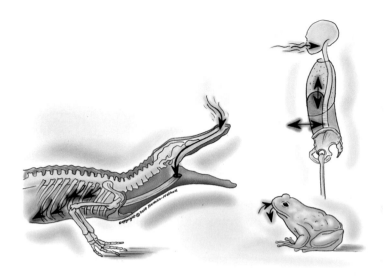

Figure I.1 Primitive air-breathing animals had to rely on swallowing movements to breathe in air.

This evolution was a great improvement over gulping air, but it came at a price. The negative pressure in the thorax not only appeared to suck in air, it also pulled the belly organs upward, and much of the space that could have been used for breathing was occupied. Primitive reptiles solved the problem by stretching a sheet of connective tissue across the bottom of the rib cage, preventing the organs from moving upward. This sheet still exists as the modern central tendon of the diaphragm (figure I.2).

Mammals, who were warm blooded, needed a higher oxygen intake. Their breathing had to become more effective at drawing oxygen into the lungs with the purpose of increasing their metabolism. Having warm blood was an advantage. They did not need to live in a warm climate for the sun to

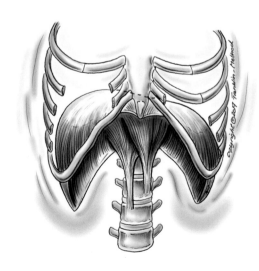

Figure I.2 The diaphragm, front view with central tendon.

heat the body until the muscles could start functioning; the body could warm itself even in a cold environment.

Muscles were attached to the rim of the central tendon and stretched down to the lower edge of the thorax, creating a muscular dome with a tendinous roof. This diaphragm could now move downward and flatten out, allowing for a large downward expansion in the lungs and greatly increasing the capacity to absorb oxygen. In fact, resting mammals can breathe with minimal movement of the ribs. As you are reading this book—unless you are running on a treadmill—you will probably not notice much movement of the rib cage. This kind of breathing, called *abdominal breathing,* probably explains why mammals lack ribs below the 12th thoracic vertebra. As you inhale, the organs below the diaphragm are pushed downward by the descending diaphragm. The abdominal wall moves outward to accommodate their movement, something that would not be possible with a bony wall of ribs (see figure I.3).

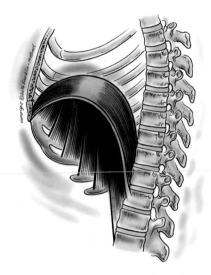

Figure I.3 The diaphragm, lateral view.

How to Use This Book

This book focuses on improving breathing function to benefit your health and improve your performance in the chores of daily life and during exercise. You will learn the anatomy of breathing and practice 35 exercises. The exercises are a combination of movement, imagery, and self-touch to create the maximum positive impact on your breathing.

The book begins by teaching you about the vital muscle of breathing: the diaphragm. Next, you will learn about the interaction of the diaphragm and the abdominal and other muscles associated with breathing, such as the scalenes. You will learn and experience the movement of the rib cage as it pertains to breathing. Finally, you will integrate all the elements involved in breathing, including the lungs and inner organs for optimal breathing function. Performing the exercises in this book will leave you feeling more energetic and focused, yet relaxed. You will also gain an understanding of how to integrate imagery into your breathing practice.

After you have read the book, choose two or three of the exercises that felt most beneficial to you and practice them for a few minutes every day. A recommended daily practice is also presented at the end of this book.

Now it's time to explore, exercise, and embody the physical apparatus involved in the act of breathing.

DIAPHRAGM

The diaphragm is a muscular dome that extends along the bottom of the rib cage. In doing so, it separates the thoracic from the abdominal cavity. It is shaped like a boomerang with a flat tendon at its center (figure 1.1).

The diaphragm is unique among muscles in that it is under both voluntary and automatic control. You do not have to consciously initiate each breath; this task would be laborious and even dangerous since you could forget to do it. The only other muscles that function similarly are the scalenes, which keep the first two ribs from dropping downward during inhalation.

Anteriorly the muscle fibers of the diaphragm insert into the bottom of the sternum at a point called the xyphoid process. Laterally the diaphragm inserts into the inner margins of the lowest six ribs. Posteriorly the diaphragm connects to the bodies of L1 and L2 (L = lumbar vertebra). This connection is provided by vertically lying muscles called the right and left crura (plural of *crus*, which is Latin for "shin" or "leg;" named for their leglike shape).

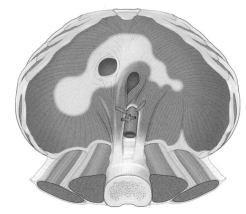

Figure 1.1 Diaphragm, view from below.

When the diaphragm is at rest, the top of its central tendon lies in front of vertebra T8 or T9 (T = thoracic). In deep inhalation it can move as far down as T11. The ventral attachment of the diaphragm is to the sternum, while the back of the diaphragm reaches all the way down to the 12th rib as well as the lumbar vertebrae. This attachment pattern causes the dorsal part of the diaphragm to be sloped steeply downward.

The two lungs sit on top of the right and left hemispheres of the diaphragm and flank the heart. The central tendon of the diaphragm blends with the pericardium, a connective tissue sack that covers the heart. During inhalation the heart is carried downward, and during expiration it is carried upward, as if it were traveling in an elevator. This constant change in position moves and stretches the heart and contributes to good circulation.

The dome of the diaphragm is higher on the right than the left. On the right side the liver, which is large and dense, displaces the diaphragm upward. On the left the stomach, which is smaller and hollow, is located below the diaphragm. At the back, tucked under the ribs and contacting the diaphragm is the spleen. Both kidneys are located just below the diaphragm. Like the heart, they are carried downward and upward by the diaphragm's movement. In total the kidneys move about 500 yards (457 m) a day, compelled by the diaphragm. Figure 1.2 shows the relationship between the diaphragm and surrounding organs.

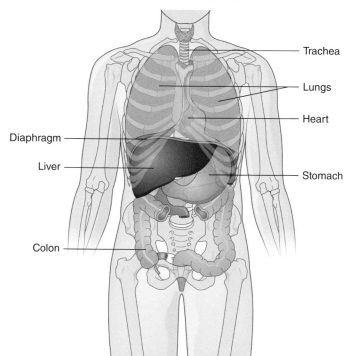

Figure 1.2 The diaphragm in relation to other anatomical structures.

The organs located below the diaphragm do not move much when you breathe lightly. During the initial phase of inhalation they are merely compressed, like a sponge. At this moment the elastic resistance of the organs helps to tone the diaphragm. During further inhalation they move downward and also escape sideways. This is why your belly moves forward and also laterally during inhalation. The location of the spine limits backward movement of the diaphragm. However, the spine does contribute to breathing by extending slightly during inhalation. The pelvic floor also adjusts to the rhythms of your breath. It moves downward during inhalation and upward during exhalation (figure 1.3).

Note that the expanding movements of the abdominal muscles and pelvic floor during inhalation are not a relaxation that needs to be inhibited at all costs. In fact, the tone in these muscles increases by about 20 percent to resist the downward fall of the organs. Holding the belly inward during inhalation comes at the cost of inhibiting the natural abdominal toning action that inhalation provides.

The aorta, vena cava, and esophagus run vertically between the thorax and the abdomen, which means they have to pass through openings in the diaphragm. The aorta passes just behind the diaphragm and in front of the vertebral column. It enters the abdomen though a tendinous arch called the median arcuate ligament. This position at the very back of the

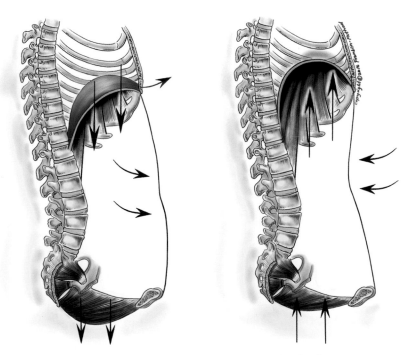

Figure 1.3 Movement of the pelvic floor in relation to the diaphragm.

diaphragm limits any squeezing of the aorta through the contractions of the diaphragm during breathing. However, intra-abdominal pressure can affect the aorta from the front.

The vena cava passes through the tendinous part of the diaphragm just right of the midline. This position outside the actual muscular part of the diaphragm limits pressures on this large vessel as well. Because the central tendon moves up and down more than most parts of the diaphragm, it has to slide along the vena cava, which is more stationary.

The esophagus lies just above the left crus and is circled by a loop of diaphragm. Surprisingly some of the fibers of this loop arise from the right crus and cross over the left just above the stomach. This design enables a sphincter action of sort during inhalation when the pressure on the stomach increases the danger of food being pushed back up again.

Two muscles, the psoas major and quadratus lumborum, pass just behind the back edge of the diaphragm. These muscles are bridged by tendinous arches, called the medial arcuate ligament and the lateral arcuate ligament. Muscle fibers of the diaphragm originate from all these tendinous arches. The fascial covering of the diaphragm is connected to the fascia of the psoas major, indicating interaction of hip flexion and breathing rhythms.

Goals for Breathing

Understanding how breathing works is the first step to exploring better breathing. The next step is to put this understanding into practice with clear goals in mind. The exercises in this book focus on creating these outcomes:

- Embodied optimal breathing function
- Improved posture
- Reduced gripping and unnecessary tension
- Improved mobility and coordination of the rib cage and thoracic spine
- Increased flexibility and strength in the muscles of breathing
- Optimized breathing patterns for individual situations
- Even movement distribution between breathing regions
- Good coordination in the powerhouse of breathing, the diaphragm
- Increased benefits of good breathing on your state of mind

Following are 13 exercises and imagery explorations for the diaphragm.

Visualizing the Diaphragm

This exercise establishes the baseline of your understanding and ability to visualize the diaphragm. Although the diaphragm is inside the body and moves up and down about 20,000 times a day, most people have trouble visualizing it. If you cannot see the design and movement of the diaphragm (or any part of the body), improving it is difficult. Positive change begins with awareness.

1. Sit or stand in a comfortable position, and do the following imagery exercise. With your eyes closed, visualize a room in your home. How many objects can you see? Can you see chairs, a table, other furniture, windows, books, and other objects? Can you see them in three dimensions and in color?

2. Now visualize your breathing diaphragm, arguably the most important muscle for your breathing (and therefore life). Can you visualize its location, shape, attachment areas, openings? Can you see it in three dimensions? Can you imagine the movement of the diaphragm?

Touching the Diaphragm

The diaphragm is attached to the bottom of the sternum at the xyphoid process, the inner margins of the lowest six ribs, and the bodies of L1 and L2 (see figure 1.3).

1. In a sitting or standing position, touch the areas where the diaphragm attaches to the skeleton. Start at the xyphoid process (at the bottom of the sternum). Imagine the diaphragm attached behind this point and sloping upward from there.

2. Slide your fingers down the rib angle from the sternum, to the right and the left. You are now feeling the inferior cartilaginous border of the rib cage where the diaphragm attaches. The diaphragm attaches to the inside of ribs 6 through 12.

3. Place your fingers between the iliac crest at the top and side of the pelvis and the lowest rib. See if you can feel a rib just above the crest. Since it's a floating rib and not attached to the sternum, it is more challenging to discover.

4. For a moment imagine the large expanse of the diaphragm, all the way from the sternum to the 12th rib.

5. Finally, touch the general area of the first and second lumbar vertebrae. Run your fingers up a few inches from the back of the pelvis to provide yourself with a general sense of the location of these vertebrae.

6. Finish by placing your fingers just below the sternum again. Cough or laugh to feel the strong contractions of the diaphragm and the abdominal wall.

Imagining the Movement of the Diaphragm

As you inhale, the diaphragm moves downward. Imagine this action as you inhale deeply. You may feel more like the diaphragm is moving upward. This sensation arises by focusing on the action of the ribs, which in fact do move upward while the diaphragm moves downward. To get started with your embodiment of breathing it is advisable to first focus on one area at a time, then later start combining the different actions into a holistic ensemble.

1. Stand or sit comfortably. Recreate the dome of the diaphragm with your hands, and place them horizontally in front of the diaphragm directly above the xyphoid process.

2. Face your palms down, and cup your hands into a dome shape to mirror the design of the diaphragm (figure 1.4).

3. To mirror the movement of the diaphragm during inhalation, move your hands downward as you inhale (figure 1.5).

4. To mirror the movement of the diaphragm during exhalation, move your hands upward as you exhale.

5. To be more precise in your imagery, you may decrease the doming of your hands as they move downward and increase it as they move upward.

6. Breathe for 5 to 10 full breath cycles while visualizing this action and mirroring it with your hands. Once you are done, you may notice that you feel calmer and your breathing has slowed down.

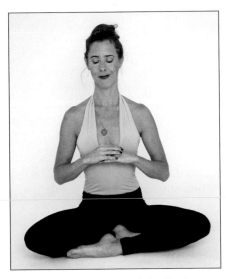

Figure 1.4 Movement of the diaphragm, starting position.

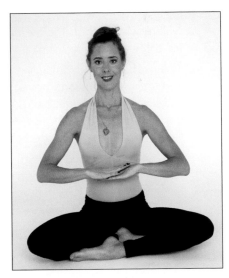

Figure 1.5 Movement of the diaphragm, inhaling.

Feeling the Movement of the Abdominal Wall

Allowing your abdominal muscles to move forward and sideways is not a letting go or relaxing of these muscles; this relaxation needs to be inhibited by pulling the navel inward. The abdominal muscles are performing an eccentric (lengthening) muscle contraction, and their tone is increasing by about 20 percent in an effort to contain the downward movement of the organs. The organ pillar provides the natural training of the abdominal muscles, and your muscles benefit from performing this eccentric contraction about 20,000 times a day. Abdominal breathing is your constant abdominal workout. There is no need to add voluntary contraction to the natural lengthening and shortening actions of the abdominal muscles. The cues that revolve around gripping your abdominals are recent inventions. Humans survived for hundreds of thousands of years without constantly needing to hold in the abdominal wall. Stabilizing the spine must happen while you keep breathing, or you will have nothing left to stabilize. The abdominal muscles can multitask and provide support for the spine while they still move for breathing.

1. Place your hands on your belly. As you inhale, notice how the abdominal wall is moving outward.

2. As you exhale, notice how the abdominal wall naturally moves back in toward the spine. Feel and visualize the movement out and in during several breathing cycles.

3. Now place your hands or the tips of your fingers on the sides of your body between the lowest ribs and the iliac crest. Feel the abdominal wall moving out during inhalation and in during exhalation. Breathe for three or four cycles to feel this action.

4. To lengthen your exhalation, exhale on a sibilant *sssss* while imagining and feeling the inward movement of the abdominal muscles. The *sssss* will slow down your exhalation and lengthen the concentric contraction of the muscle. Perform only one exhalation on *sssss*, then allow for a natural breathing cycle before repeating.

5. Once you are done, let your arms rest at your sides. Notice any changes in your posture and the overall sense of your body.

Visualizing the Interaction of the Diaphragm and Abdominal Muscles

As you inhale the diaphragm descends like a piston, displacing the organs downward, forward, and to the sides. You will use your hands to visualize the interaction between the movement of the diaphragm and the abdominal wall. You can do this exercise standing, sitting, or supine.

1. Model the dome of the diaphragm with your right (or left) hand, and place the hand horizontally in front of the diaphragm just above the xyphoid process.

2. Place your other hand in a vertical position in front your belly; this hand will mirror the movement of the abdominal wall (figure 1.6).

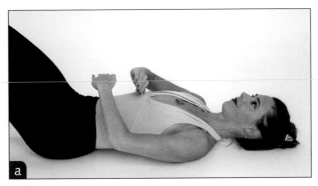

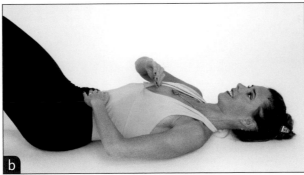

Figure 1.6 Modeling the movement of the abdominal wall and diaphragm during (a) inhalation and (b) exhalation.

(continued)

Visualizing the Interaction of the Diaphragm and Abdominal Muscles (continued)

3. The abdominal wall moves outward during inhalation and inward during exhalation. Alternatively you can also hold a prop, such as a piece of felt, to help you visualize the movements.

4. As you inhale, your diaphragm hand moves downward and your abdominal hand moves forward.

5. As you exhale, your diaphragm hand moves upward and your abdominal hand moves inward. Repeat this action three or four times.

6. Now move your abdominal hand to the side of the body between your iliac crest and the lowest ribs. Your abdominal hand will now mirror the movement of the lateral body wall. As you inhale, the diaphragm hand moves down and the abdominal hand moves laterally. As you exhale, the diaphragm hand moves upward and the abdominal hand moves inward. Repeat this action three or four times, switch hands, and perform the same modeling of the abdominal wall and diaphragm on the other side of the body wall.

7. Rest for a moment, and notice any changes in your posture and overall sense of your body. Your abdominal muscles may actually feel more alive and toned; breathing is the 24-hour workout for the abdominal wall. When you allow the movement to occur in a functional way, you actually increase the abdominal tone by emphasizing the full movement of the abdominal muscles.

Visualizing the Movement of the Pelvic Floor

The pelvic floor moves downward on inhalation and upward on exhalation. This movement reflects the downward and upward movement of the organ column. Once again, the downward movement of the pelvic floor is not a letting go; the muscle tone of the pelvic floor increases by 20 percent during its descent. The muscles of the pelvic floor are contracting eccentrically, which is strengthening and should not be inhibited by constantly holding the pelvic floor up. Here, too, the descending column of organs acts as the dumbbell to train these muscles.

1. Stand in a comfortable position. Create an inverted dome with your hands by placing your fingers on top of each other and facing your palms upward.
2. Place your hands in front of the pelvis, just below the level of the pubic symphysis.
3. Move your hands an inch or two downward during inhalation to reflect the movement of the pelvic floor during inhalation.
4. Move your hands an inch or two upward to reflect the movement of the pelvic floor during exhalation.
5. Repeat this action five or six times, rest your arms at your sides, and notice any changes in your posture and the tone of your pelvic floor.

Visualizing the Interaction of the Pelvic Floor and the Diaphragm

In this exercise you visualize the movement of the pelvic floor and diaphragm concurrently. Although both of these muscular domes move in the same direction during breathing (downward on inhalation and upward on exhalation), they perform the opposite actions during the movement. During inhalation, the muscle fibers of the diaphragm shorten while the muscles of the pelvic floor lengthen; and during exhalation, the muscle fibers of the diaphragm lengthen while the muscles of the pelvic floor shorten. In this exercise you will use your hands to model the similarity in direction of the muscles—downward and upward—while being aware that they are contracting in the opposite fashion.

1. Stand in a comfortable position. With one hand, model the diaphragm by cupping your hand and placing it in front of the lower sternum, palm facing downward. With the other hand, model the pelvic floor by placing a hand in front of the pelvis, just below the pubic symphysis with the palm facing upward. Both hands are in the transverse plane with the upper palm down and the lower palm up (figure 1.7).

2. As you inhale, both hands move downward to mirror the movement of the diaphragm and pelvic floor.

3. As you exhale, both hands move upward to mirror the movement of the pelvic floor and diaphragm.

4. Breathe for five or six full cycles while modeling the movement with your hands, then rest your arms at your sides. Notice any changes in posture and your breathing patterns.

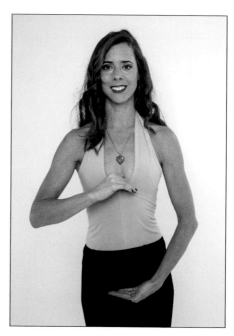

Figure 1.7 Synchronizing the movement of the diaphragm and pelvic floor with hand modeling.

Shaking the Diaphragm to Increase Circulation and Proprioception

The diaphragm needs the same skills as other muscles, namely, strength and flexibility, as well as good circulation and the ability to relax on occasion. You can improve these functions with a range of exercises. In this exercise, you will improve circulation to the diaphragm and increase sensory awareness through movement.

1. Stand in a comfortable position. Reach your right arm forward, then shake and jiggle it. Imagine the muscles of your arm to be floppy and flexible. Imagine the muscles of your arms to be loose cloth fluttering in the wind.

2. Now let your right arm rest at your side, and notice how it feels in comparison to your left arm. You may be aware of a greater sense of relaxation and flexibility in your right arm. Stretch both arms forward and upward, and compare their ease of movement and flexibility. You may notice that the right arm feels more mobile and flexible. Repeat this exercise with your left arm.

3. Now that you are aware of how jiggling the arm improves flexibility, circulation, and sensation, do the same thing with the diaphragm. The challenge here is that the muscles of the diaphragm are inside the rib cage, whereas in the arm the muscles are on the outside of the bones.

4. Shake and jiggle your rib cage. Make an *aaaaa* sound as you shake. The sound will help you hear and sense whether your diaphragm is moving in response to your jiggle.

5. Rest for a moment, and repeat the shaking and jiggling of the rib cage. Try different sounds, such as *ooooo* or *eeeee*.

6. Now add some shaking of your arms and shoulders as you shake your rib cage and diaphragm.

7. Rest your arms at your sides, and notice any changes in your posture and breathing. You may notice that your breathing is deeper and fuller and that your posture has improved.

Imagining the Diaphragm as a Trampoline

In the following exercise you will loosen the diaphragm while performing small jumps. It is a great way to release tension in the diaphragm and increase its movement potential.

1. Stand in a comfortable position. Imagine your diaphragm to be a flexible trampoline stretched out at the bottom of the rib cage. The heart and lung are perched on top of this trampoline.
2. Perform small hops up and down, while making a *ha* sound every time you land on your feet. Imagine the diaphragm moving in sync with the sound.
3. Perform the jumping and *ha* sound while visualizing the trampoline bouncing up and down for about 15 seconds.

Stretching Your Diaphragm

The diaphragm needs its own designated stretching and strengthening routine, just like any other muscle. The diaphragm moves downward when you inhale, expanding the lungs and creating a vacuum. This vacuum causes air to rush into the lungs and oxygen to transfer through the thin walls of the lungs into the bloodstream. (For more information on the lungs, see chapter 2.)

What makes the diaphragm move downward? The diaphragm is a muscle, and muscles can shorten and lengthen between the origin and the insertion of the muscle. The origin is considered the fixed point, while the insertion is the part that is moved by the muscle.

If you want to stretch the diaphragm, you need to increase the distance between the origin and insertion, as in the following exercise. This exercise stretches other muscles, such as the intercostals (between the ribs) and the oblique abdominals, which in turn increases the benefit for the diaphragm.

1. Stand in a comfortable position. You will begin by stretching the left side of the diaphragm. These fibers are mostly located between the 12th rib and the central tendon along the inside of the rib cage, which is called the zone of opposition. Lift your left arm over your head, and place your right hand on your lower ribs on the left side (figure 1.8).

2. As you exhale, laterally flex your spine to the right (figure 1.9). Two factors are causing the diaphragm to lengthen as you perform this movement—the fact that you are exhaling, and the increase in distance between the 12th rib and the top of the diaphragm.

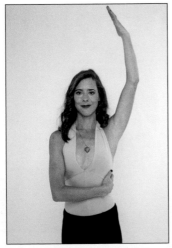

Figure 1.8 Diaphragm stretch, starting position.

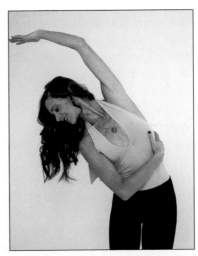

Figure 1.9 Exhaling with lateral flexion of the spine to stretch the diaphragm.

(continued)

Stretching Your Diaphragm *(continued)*

3. Inhale as you return to the upright position. Repeat the movement for five breath cycles. Exhale as you move to the right; inhale as you return to the upright position.

4. Imagine the muscle fibers of the diaphragm lengthening underneath your ribs. To increase the stretch, gently push down on the left lower ribs (7-12) with your right hand.

5. Return your left arm to the side of the body and rest for a moment. Notice any differences between the two sides of the body. The entire right side of your body may feel more relaxed. Imagine breathing into your right lung, then your left lung. Does it feel as if your right lung takes in much more air than the left? That is because the right hemisphere got stretched and is more flexible, allowing for more movement of the diaphragm and ribs.

6. Perform the same exercise on the other side. Lift your right arm up above your head, place your left hand on the right side of the rib cage, and flex your spine to the left while exhaling. Repeat the movement for five cycles of breath. As you move to the left, exhale; as you return to the upright position, inhale.

7. To finish the exercise, reach up with both arms and clasp your hands. Laterally flex your spine to the right and left (figure 1.10). During lateral flexion, exhale; when you return to center, inhale. Move to the right and left four times.

8. Drop your arms down to your sides, and rest in the standing position for a moment. You may notice that your posture has improved, your lungs feel as though they are lifting you upward like balloons, and your sternum is higher. Working with your breath is good for your posture and general sense of well-being.

9. Be aware of the stretch of the diaphragm when you exercise. Notice how movement of the thorax and spine affect the length of the fibers of the diaphragm. Use this awareness to increase the stretching of your diaphragm, even when you are focusing also on other aspects of the exercise.

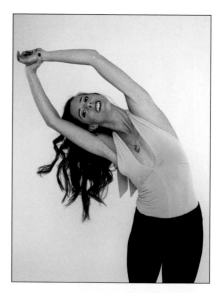

Figure 1.10 Laterally flex to the right, exhale in lateral flexion, and inhale as you move to the center position.

Exhaling on *SSSSS* or Through a Straw to Lengthen the Exhalation

When you focus on lengthening your exhalation, you can simultaneously increase your capacity for inhalation and calm down. The exhalation is the calming phase of the breath cycle, which is generally divided into inhalation, exhalation, and a short pause. This exercise requires a straw.

1. Take a natural inhalation, and exhale on a sibilant *sssss*.
2. Take a few natural breaths without the *sssss*.
3. Once again, inhale and exhale on *sssss*.
4. Notice whether your natural breathing has calmed down and become slower.
5. Put a straw between your lips. Gently blow through the straw until you have fully exhaled. Do not use any extra effort, and do not force the exhalation.
6. Take a natural inhalation.
7. Repeat the exhalation through the straw and inhalation without the straw for a few more cycles of breath.
8. Pause, remove the straw, and notice changes in your state of mind. You may now feel calmer and more relaxed.

Strengthening Your Diaphragm

In this exercise, you will challenge the diaphragm by adding some abdominal movement. You should perform this exercise after you are proficient at the previous version.

1. Lift your right arm over your head, and place your left hand on your lower ribs on the right side. Laterally flex your spine to the left as you exhale.

2. Remaining in this laterally flexed position, consciously breathe in and out three times. Focus on the movement of the diaphragm and abdominal wall. Every time you exhale, allow the lateral flexion to slightly increase. It should happen naturally, just by feeling the weight of your body.

3. Once you have done three cycles of breath, use the next inhalation to initiate your movement back to the upright position. Focus on the diaphragm on the inside of the rib cage, rather than the abdominal muscles, doing the job.

4. Repeat this sequence on the other side. Lift your left arm up above your head, place your right hand on the left side of the rib cage, and flex your spine to the right while exhaling.

5. Remain in this laterally flexed position and consciously breathe in and out three times for three full cycles. Every time you exhale, allow the lateral flexion of your body to increase.

6. Use the inhalation to bring you back to the upright position. Focus on the diaphragm on the inside of the rib cage.

7. Once you are done, rest in the standing position for a moment. You may notice that your posture has improved and your spine has lengthened naturally. Most likely your breathing is deeper and your shoulders are relaxed.

8. To increase the challenge for your diaphragm, you can also perform this exercise with a book in your hand or a 1-pound (0.45 kg) dumbbell.

Lengthening Your Diaphragm

In this exercise, you will use a metaphor to improve the length and strength of your diaphragm. Imagery in the form of metaphors has a training effect that is not unlike performing a physical exercise.

1. Stand in a comfortable position and follow your inhalations and exhalations for three cycles.
2. As you exhale, imagine a floating balloon beneath your diaphragm. Imagine this balloon assisting the upward movement of the diaphragm, allowing the muscle fibers to stretch more fully.
3. As you inhale, imagine a soft pillow resting on the top of diaphragm, allowing it to move downward (figure 1.11).
4. Inhale and exhale five times with the balloon and pillow image.
5. Rest your mind, breathe naturally, and notice any changes in your breathing.

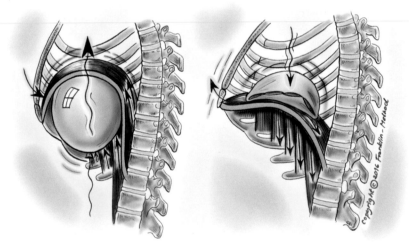

Figure 1.11 In this image, a balloon lifts the diaphragm on exhalation and a pillow helps to move downward on inhalation

RIB CAGE

The thoracic wall consists of 12 ribs, the thoracic spine, the sternum, and an array of articulations, muscles, and ligaments. The interaction of these parts is complex, and it is important for breathing, spinal stability, and movement. The thoracic wall can flexibly expand due to the articulation of its ribs with other parts of the body wall by true joints. The shape and the orientation of the ribs (figure 2.1) contribute to the expansion of the thorax.

The ribs attach posteriorly to the thoracic spine and anteriorly to costal cartilages. All ribs connect to the spinal column, but only the upper seven connect via their cartilages to the sternum; they are called the true ribs. The remaining pairs of ribs are called false ribs. The costal cartilages of ribs 7 to 10 connect with the costal cartilages of the ribs above them, whereas ribs 11 and 12 have no anterior connection. This arrangement allows the inferior part of the rib cage to be more flexible and adaptive to the movement of the diaphragm and organs.

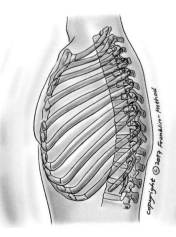

Figure 2.1 The rib cage, lateral view.

The ribs are the most flexible bones in the body. They consist of a curved and a slightly spiraled shaft. The part of the rib that connects to the spine is characterized by a head, a neck, and a tubercle (figure 2.2). You can metaphorically visualize the head, neck, and tubercle of the rib as a foot in a slipper. The heel is the tubercle, the head is the ball of the foot and the toes, and the arch of the foot is the neck of the rib.

There are usually two articulations—the costovertebral and the costotransverse joints—that connect the ribs to the spine. The costovertebral joint is formed by the head of the rib connecting into a facet formed by two vertebral bodies, its own, and the one above it. Ribs 1, 11, and 12 articulate only with their respective vertebrae. The costo-

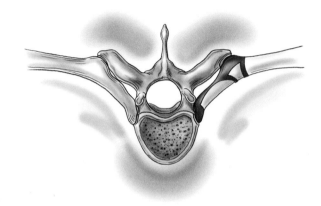

Figure 2.2 Head, neck, and tubercle of rib compared to a foot.

transverse joints are formed by the tubercle of the rib connecting to a corresponding facet on the transverse process of the associated vertebra.

During inhalation, the backs of the ribs rotate and slide down in their respective joints while the shafts of the ribs rotate upward (figure 2.3).

The angle formed between the two joints determines the movement of the individual rib. The costovertebral joints (CV) 9 through 12 are shifted posteriorly, creating the more lateral bucket-handle movement (figure 2.4).

The first to seventh ribs connect to the cartilage around the sternum, which connects to the sternum itself, called the chondrosternal joints. They are synovial joints, which have some ability to rotate and slide during

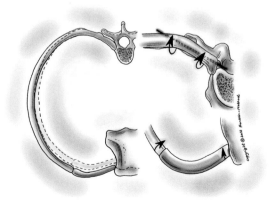

Figure 2.3 Rotation of the ribs during inhalation.

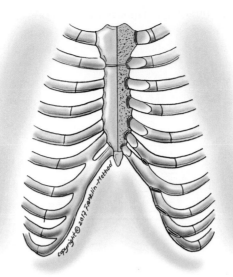

Figure 2.4 Rib cage, anterior view with costal cartilages and costosternal joints.

breathing and movement. The connection of costal cartilage of the first rib to the sternum is fibrocartilaginous, creating the firm connection between the movement of the first rib and the sternum.

The body of the sternum is flat and slightly curved forward (figure 2.5). The joints between the body of the sternum and the xyphoid process usually form a symphysis. Only slight movement is possible in these joints during breathing, but maintaining this flexibility throughout your life is important.

The posterior attachment of the ribs to the spine is generally superior to the anterior attachment. Therefore, when a rib elevates, it moves the anterior thoracic wall forward relative to the

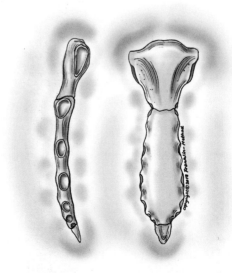

Figure 2.5 The sternum.

posterior wall, a movement like the lifting of a pump handle (figure 2.6a). The middle part of each rib is inferior to its two ends. When this region of the ribs is elevated, it expands the thoracic wall laterally.

This movement is like the lifting of a bucket handle (figure 2.6b). The inferior two ribs are not attached to cartilage in front; they simply move backward like the opening of a caliper (figure 2.6c).

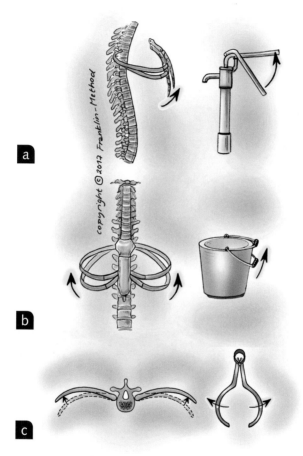

Figure 2.6 Movement of the ribs is like lifting (a) a pump handle, (b) a bucket handle, and (c) a caliper.

The first two ribs are flat, and they lie close to the horizontal plane in an upright position. Their action is mostly of the pump handle type, while the ribs in the middle of the thorax move more laterally. A slouched posture tends to lower all ribs anteriorly and reduce their ability to increase the volume within the thoracic wall.

Because the ribs have some ability to move forward, laterally, and backward and the diaphragm moves downward on inhalation, the lungs can be expanded in a three-dimensional fashion during inhalation (figure 2.7). During quiet breathing, the movement of the diaphragm dominates; during deeper breathing, the movements of the rib cage become more prominent.

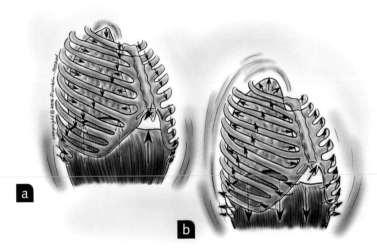

Figure 2.7 Three-dimensional expansion of the rib cage and downward movement to the diaphragm during *(a)* exhalation and *(b)* inhalation.

Following are five exercises and imagery explorations for the rib cage.

Three-Dimensional Thoracic Movement

In this exercise, you will focus on the three-dimensional movement of the rib cage during breathing.

1. Start this exercise in an upright sitting or a comfortable standing position. Place your hands on the sternum; one hand is on top of the other. As you take a deep breath, notice how the sternum moves upward and forward. This is the pump-handle component of your thoracic breathing.

2. Place one hand each on the sides of the middle section of your rib cage. As you inhale, notice how these ribs move laterally. Imagine them as the handles of a bucket that are moving up during inhalation and down during exhalation.

3. Place your hands on the lowest ribs, just above the pelvis. As you take a deep inhalation, feel how the lowest ribs move posteriorly. Imagine ribs 11 and 12 widening and moving backward into your hands when you inhale and forward again when you exhale.

4. Finally, imagine the combination of these three movements—to the front, side, and back. As you inhale, imagine the movement forward to the front, side, and back; as you exhale, imagine the reverse movements.

5. During your sport or exercise practice, focus on using three-dimensional breathing in your rib cage rather than focusing on only one dimension.

Imagery for Releasing Tension in the Rib Cage

Imagery that facilitates the flexibility of the ribs and the ease of their movement will improve your breathing capacity. The best metaphors are often the ones you discover yourself. This exercise provides two examples to get you started.

1. Stand or sit in a comfortable position and imagine tiny balloons attached to the shafts of your ribs.

2. As you inhale, these balloons help to lift your ribs upward (figure 2.8). As you exhale the balloons release their pull and the ribs float back down.

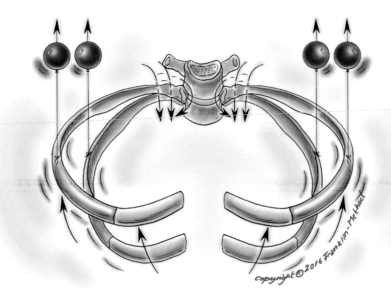

Figure 2.8 Image of tiny balloons lifting the ribs upward.

(continued)

Imagery for Releasing Tension in the Rib Cage *(continued)*

3. Imagine your rib cage as a soft cloth suspended from your first rib (figure 2.9).

4. As you inhale, the cloth swings outward; as you exhale, it drops back again.

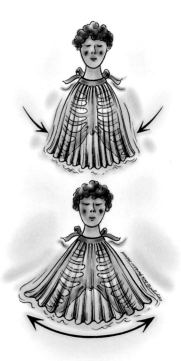

Figure 2.9 Image of the rib cage as a soft cloth.

Elastic Sternum and Rib Cartilages

The sternum and their adjoining joints and cartilages need to slide, move, and twist as you breathe. In this exercise, you use imagery and touch to facilitate these actions.

1. Sit upright or stand in a comfortable position. Place one hand on the manubrium and the other on the body of the sternum.
2. As you flex and extend your spine, imagine the small and subtle movement at the manubriosternal symphysis.
3. Touch the joints between the cartilage and bone on the left and right side of your sternum. They may feel a bit tender.
4. As you inhale and exhale, imagine slight sliding and rotating movement at these joints.
5. Imagine cartilage performing a slight spiraling action as the ribs rotate up and down during breathing.
6. With your fingers on the cartilages, perform spinal flexion, extension, lateral flexion, and rotation, and feel how the cartilage adapts to both movement and breathing.
7. Remove your touch, and notice changes in your posture and breathing. Most likely your sternum will feel as if it is naturally more lifted and it will be easier to breathe in the front-to-back dimension.

Down in Back, Up in Front

During inhalation, the ribs rotate posteriorly in their costovertebral and costotransverse articulation. This means that the backs of the ribs are moving down, while the fronts are moving up (see figure 2.3).

1. Sit upright or stand and visualize how your ribs connect to your spine.
2. As you inhale, visualize the movement of the ribs. They are rotating posteriorly in their costovertebral and costotransverse joints; the backs of the ribs are actually moving down.
3. Imagine this down-the-back feeling facilitating the up-in-front action of the ribs. If you focus on the whole rib moving up on inhalation, it will actually impede your breathing.

Tapping the Rib Cage

With the help of your hands or a pair of balls, you can loosen the rib cage and create more elasticity in the intercostal muscles. For this example, use orange Franklin Method balls or simply make loose fists with your hands.

1. Sit or stand in a comfortable position.
2. Tap the right side of your rib cage with your loose fists or two balls (figure 2.10).
3. Flex to the side as you tap, rotate your spine as you tap, then flex and extend your spine as you tap.
4. After a minute of tapping, rest for a moment. Compare the breathing and rib motion of the right and left sides.
5. Repeat the tapping on the other side.

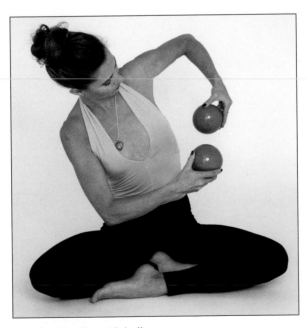

Figure 2.10   Tapping the ribs with balls.

LUNGS

Located in the chest cavity, the lungs are two large organs of respiration and ventilation. They are responsible for aerating the blood. Ventilation is the process of bringing air into the lungs, and respiration is the process of gas exchange in the lungs. During the process of respiration, oxygen passes into the bloodstream while carbon dioxide is removed from the blood.

Breathing with lungs comes with a few challenges. The airways must be kept sufficiently patent, the air must be 100 percent moisturized, and the lungs require constant cleaning from dust and other particles. Because air pressure is much lower than water pressure, land animals have a very large and thin surface for gas exchange to facilitate passage of oxygen into the blood. If you were to spread out the inner surface of the lungs, the size of this surface would approximate a tennis court.

The lungs are located inside the rib cage and sit on top of the two hemispheres of the diaphragm (figure 3.1). Between them

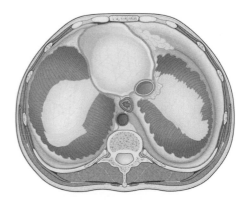

Figure 3.1 View of the diaphragm from above. The heart rests on the area occupied by the central tendon, while the lungs sit on the right and left costal diaphragm.

lie the heart and other structures within the mediastinum (the area containing the heart and great vessels).

The lungs follow the movement of the diaphragm and rib cage due to the vacuum that exists between the two structures. Each lung is encased in a thin membranous sac called the visceral pleura. The visceral pleura is intimately connected but continuous with the parietal pleura (figure 3.2). The parietal pleura lies along the inside of the thoracic wall, the diaphragm, and the mediastinum.

The visceral and parietal pleura can slide on top of each other due to a thin film of fluid between them. No ligaments or muscles directly attach to the lung; doing so would damage the lung and limit the amount of available movement.

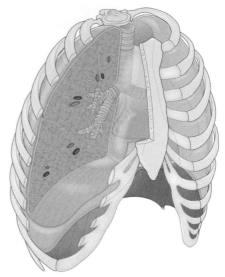

Figure 3.2 Parietal and visceral pleura surrounding the lungs.

During inhalation, the rib cage and diaphragm pull the parietal pleura outward, which in turn tugs on the visceral pleura, making the lungs expand and slide into the available space. The surface between the parietal and visceral pleura can be considered the largest joint in the body, permitting both the movements of breathing and any movement relating to the adjustments of the thorax and spine.

A common misconception about breathing is that the lungs expand similarly to the blowing up of a balloon during inhalation. The reverse is true. The lungs are not expanded by pressure increasing on the inside but by the vacuum that surrounds them.

To create a model of this mechanism, cover a glass with a flexible membrane. Two balloons (the lungs) are stuck inside the glass with their openings to the outside of the container. If you pull the membrane downward, a negative pressure is created around the balloons, expanding them outward as air rushes into the balloons (figure 3.3). It is important to keep both the rib cage and diaphragm strong and flexible in order to make sure the lungs can be stretched and moved on a regular basis to remain pliant.

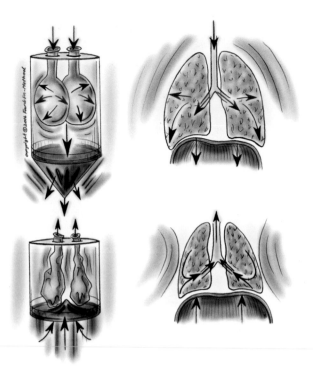

Figure 3.3 Model for understanding lung expansion.

Each lung is divided into lobes separated from one another by a tissue fissure. The right lung has three major lobes; the left lung, which is slightly smaller because of the asymmetrical placement of the heart, has two lobes. Internally, each lobe further subdivides into hundreds of lobules. Each lobule contains a bronchiole and affiliated branches, a thin wall, and clusters of alveoli. These lobes need to be able to slide on top of each other during respiration and during movements of the torso. Lack of exercise and poor posture contribute to reduced mobility in the lobes as well as the whole lung within the thorax impeding full breathing. In the example of a yoga asana in figure 3.4 we can see the necessity of having mobility in the lobes of the lung and the organs adjoining the diaphragm.

Alveoli are the tiny air sacs in which the actual gas exchange takes place. Each lung contains about 480,000 alveoli, which is one reason the inner surface of the lung is so large.

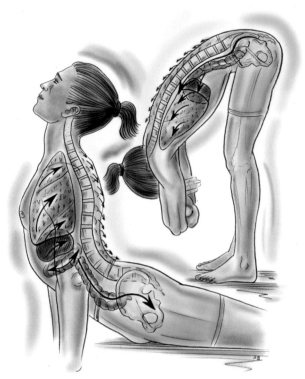

Figure 3.4 The lungs moving in a yoga asana.

The alveoli are covered by surfactant to reduce the surface tension created by the thin film of water inside them. As you inhale, much of the resistance to the expansion of the lungs stems from this surface tension within the lungs. Inhalation is further resisted by the elastic tissue of the lung and by any lack of compliancy in the joints, fascia, and muscle of the rib cage and diaphragm.

Good posture is essential to good lung function; if you slouch, the lungs will simply not be able to expand fully (figure 3.5). In addition, the lungs will become less flexible and lose some of their elasticity. Because the heart sits on the diaphragm and between the lungs, it is also negatively affected by slouched posture.

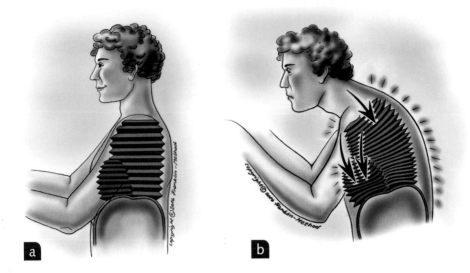

Figure 3.5 Posture and the heart and lungs: *(a)* good posture and *(b)* slouched posture.

Following are six exercises and imagery explorations for the lungs.

Lungs, Pleura, and Rib Cage

It may feel as though the filling of lungs with air is what expands them, but the reverse is true. In fact, the lungs are pulled outward by the rib cage and diaphragm creating a vacuum in the lungs, drawing the air in. In this exercise, you will embody how the lungs are pulled into expansion by the surrounding vacuum.

1. In a comfortable upright sitting or standing position, imagine the lungs inside your rib cage sitting on the diaphragm.

2. As you inhale, imagine the diaphragm pulling the lungs downward while the ribs pull the lungs forward, sideways, and to the back.

3. To embody how this works, try imagery such as the syringe or the bellows. The bellows is widened to draw the air in by creating a slight vacuum within it. In the case of the syringe, the sliding plunger represents the moving diaphragm. Pulling upward on the plunger to create suction represents the inhale; pushing it down represents the exhale.

4. Exhalation is more passive, powered by the recoil of the lungs, muscles, and associated fascia. Unless you are in the supine position, the abdominal wall will actively assist in exhalation.

5. Inhale again, and imagine the sequence of events that expand the lungs: The rib cage moves outward and pulls on the parietal pleura; the parietal pleura pulls on the visceral pleura; and the visceral pleura expands the lungs.

6. During exhalation, this sequence reverses: The lungs recoil, pulling the pleura and rib cage inward.

Costodiaphragmatic Recess

Visualizing how and where the lungs move when you inhale helps improve your breathing. The lungs expand outward during inhalation, but they also slide into available space between folded layers of parietal pleura. One of the largest of these layers lies between the lowest ribs and the back of the diaphragm at the junction of the costal and diaphragmatic pleura. This area is called the costodiaphragmatic recess.

1. In a comfortable upright sitting or standing position, place your hands on the back and bottom of the rib cage, and visualize the area between the ribs and the diaphragm.

2. As you inhale, imagine the lungs sliding into this area. They are opening the space between two folds of parietal pleura—one covering the diaphragm, the other covering the inside of the rib cage.

3. Compare the feeling to sliding your hands into a glove. As you exhale, the lungs slide out of this area and the costal and diaphragmatic pleura close.

4. Inhale and exhale several times, and imagine the lungs sliding into the costodiaphragmatic recess (figure 3.6). Use the metaphor of sliding your hands into gloves to help you with embodying this anatomical function.

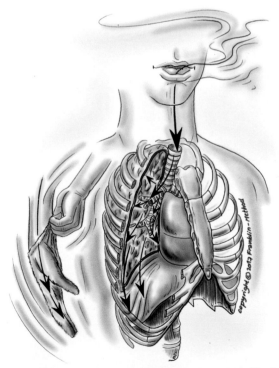

Figure 3.6 Lungs sliding into the costodiaphragmatic recess like hands into gloves.

Lungs as Sponges

The lungs can be compared to large sponges that can fill with air by expanding and empty themselves of air by contracting. It is important to practice exhaling as much air as possible to increase the elasticity of the lungs.

1. In a comfortable upright sitting or standing position, place your fingertips on your right and left shoulders; the elbows are pointing to the sides.

2. Exhale rapidly while moving your elbows and arms forward and flexing your spine. Imagine the lungs as sponges, squeezing out their air.

3. As you inhale, slowly extend your spine and move your arms and elbows back again. Imagine the lungs as sponges, filling with fresh air.

4. Match the movement with your natural breathing capacity; do not overly force your exhalation or inhalation.

5. Repeat the sequence four or five times. Repeat the movement two or three more times, but this time as you inhale, focus on the expansive power of the thorax and diaphragm. As you exhale, focus on the elastic recoil of the lungs.

Spiraling Lungs

As you inhale, the lungs not only expand but also rotate slightly outward. This rotation occurs because of the movement of the ribs and the diaphragm. Imagining this action will free your lungs and lead to deeper and fuller breathing.

1. In a comfortable upright sitting or standing position place both your hands on your right lung; the left hand is on the lower part, and the right hand is on the upper part (figure 3.7). As you inhale, imagine the outward rotation of the lungs. Support the action by slowly sliding your hands laterally on your rib cage.

2. As you exhale, imagine the lungs rotating internally. Support the action by slowly sliding your hands medially on your rib cage.

3. Repeat the breathing imagery and touch three times. Remove your hands, and compare the breathing capacity of the two lungs. Inhale into the lung on the side you practiced, then inhale into the other lung. You may notice that the lung you practiced with is more flexible and can breathe more fully than the other.

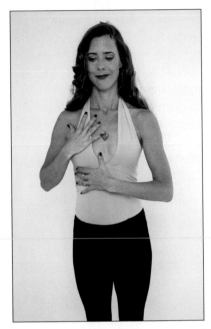

Figure 3.7 Supporting the lateral rotation of the lungs with your hands.

4. Repeat the exercise on the other side.

5. Finally, imagine both lungs at the same time. As you inhale, they expand in all directions but also move laterally; the right lung moves to the right, the left lung to the left. Imagine the movement as two cogwheels moving in opposite directions.

Expanding the Tops of the Lungs

The tops of the lungs with the pleura are higher up than you may think. They go beyond the first rib and are behind the clavicle. Ligaments connect the pleura to the first rib and the cervical spine (figure 3.8). These connections keep the lungs from being pulled down during inhalation. In this exercise, you aim to experience your breathing in this area as well.

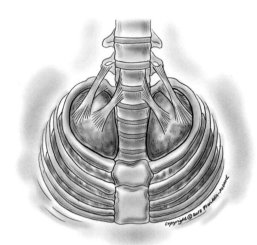

Figure 3.8 Ligaments connecting the pleura to the first rib and cervical spine.

1. In an upright sitting or comfortable standing position place your right hand on your left shoulder. Your thumb should be touching your neck (figure 3.9).

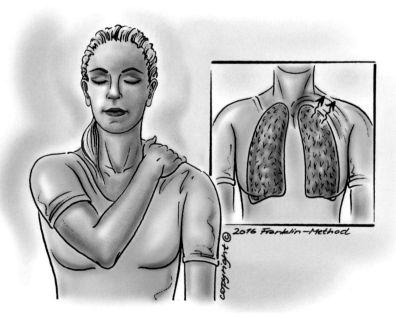

Figure 3.9 Breathing into the tops of the lungs.

2. Imagine the pleura below your touch. As you inhale deeply, imagine the lungs reaching up into this area as they expand. The lungs are moving up beyond the top rib.

3. As you exhale, imagine the lungs moving down again.

4. For several breath cycles, imagine the lungs expanding into this area adjacent your neck.

5. Remove your hand, and rest your arms at your sides. Breathe into both lungs, and notice any differences in breathing capacity. You may also notice that the left shoulder has relaxed.

6. Repeat the exercise on the other side.

Supine Breathing Practice

The supine position facilitates breathing. Because gravity is not pulling the organs downward as in the standing position, exhalation is facilitated. In this exercise, you use this fact to lengthen your exhalation and create deeper, calmer breathing. Lengthening your exhalation increases the parasympathetic activity of the autonomic nervous system. This leads to a state of relaxation and regeneration.

1. Lie comfortably on the floor in a supine position. You can stretch out your legs or bend your knees to 90 degrees.

2. Visualize the important structures of breathing: the rib cage, the lungs, the diaphragm, and the abdominal muscles.

3. Feel how gravity is acting on your rib cage and lungs. Allow the right lung to rest in the right rib cage, the left lung in the left rib cage.

4. Imagine the diaphragm moving down as you inhale. Feel how the abdominal wall moves outward (upward) during this phase.

5. Imagine the diaphragm moving upward as you exhale. Feel how the abdominal wall moves inward (drops down) toward the spine during exhalation.

6. Notice any other areas in your body where you may experience breathing. Notice your pelvic floor and movement in your rib cage.

7. Imagine your rib cage to be very flexible for breathing. As you exhale, imagine your rib cage dropping downward like a soft piece of cloth.

8. During exhalation, also imagine the lengthening of the muscle fibers of the diaphragm.

9. Exhale on a sibilant *sssss* to lengthen your exhalation.

10. Take a few natural breaths, then repeat the *sssss*.

11. Notice whether your breathing has become slower, calmer, and freer.

12. Take your time to rise to a standing position, and aim to maintain full and free breathing in your daily activities and exercise practice.

MUSCLES OF BREATHING

Any muscle that attaches to the thorax can potentially assist with breathing. Many of these muscles are involved in the movement of the upper and lower extremities as well as stabilization of the spine and thorax. These muscles only come into play during increased exertion or forced breathing. If you take a deep breath as you are reading this text, you are using some of these accessory muscles.

Primary and Accessory Muscles of Breathing

Muscles involved in quiet breathing are the diaphragm, scalenes, and intercostals. The diaphragm is the most important muscle of the group. It provides 60 to 80 percent of the breathing power through its ability to increase the volume of the rib cage in three dimensions.

The diaphragm is the first muscle to be activated during inspiration. Initially the contraction of the diaphragm causes its dome to descend and flatten. This descent is possible only because the inferior ribs are being held downward toward the pelvis by the quadratus lumborum muscle. If this were not the case, contraction of the diaphragm would pull the inferior ribs upward and the dome of the diaphragm would not descend.

At a certain point during inspiration intra-abdominal pressure, resistance of the abdominal muscles, and elasticity of the thoracic contents stop the descent of the diaphragm. The continued contraction of the diaphragm now serves to lift the six lower ribs. Intra-abdominal pressure also pushes the lower ribs and rib cartilages outward, providing circumferential expansion of the basal rib cage.

Abdominal Muscles and Breathing

The body wall extends from the first rib down to the pelvic floor. The rib cage provides strong reinforcement and stability in the thoracic area, while the pelvis provides a stable ring at the inferior end of the spine. The body wall in between these two areas is made of the abdominal muscles and associated fascia (figure 4.1).

This lack of bony restrictions in the lumbar area enables breathing with a diaphragm, which requires a flexible abdominal wall. It also helps to lengthen your stride, because the pelvis is freed up to swing and rotate, assisting your legs in swinging forward. Breathing and gait are intimately connected through these mechanisms.

The four abdominal muscles are the rectus abdominis (RA), the external and internal obliques (EO; IO), and the transversus abdominis (TA). They need to fulfill many simultaneous functions, such as breathing, stability, force absorption, load transfer, and movement. No matter what type of exercise or training you are doing, these activities need to be controlled in a balanced and efficient manner.

The EO and IO both serve to depress the ribs in a forced exhalation. They are rotators of the spine and contract eccentrically during inhalation. The TA is the largest muscle in the body, performing many simultaneous tasks. It originates in the back by the posterior and anterior

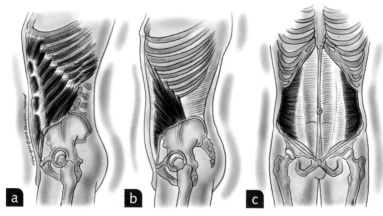

Figure 4.1 Abdominal muscles: *(a)* external obliques, *(b)* internal obliques, and *(c)* transversus abdominis.

layer of the thoracolumbar fascia (TLF). The upper TA interdigitates with the diaphragm, indicating its intimate function in breathing. The TA functions as a contractile tube surrounding the abdominal viscera. It works antagonistically with the diaphragm to help the organs move inward and upward during exhalation in all but the supine position. The TA is a stabilizer of the lumbar spine through its connections to the TLF. Its fascia splits into the sheaths that surround the erector spinae. Anteriorly it forms the posterior wall of the rectus sheath. The TA effectively can reinforce the posterior and anterior body wall while it participates in breathing (figure 4.2).

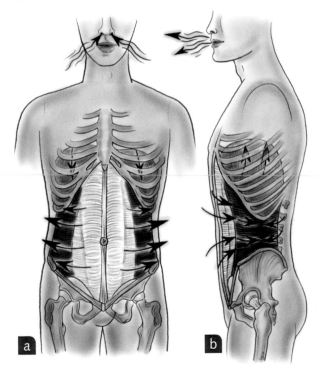

Figure 4.2 Transversus abdominis (TA) during *(a)* inspiration and *(b)* expiration.

The Core and Breathing

The four classic muscles of core stability are the transversus abdominis (TA), the diaphragm, the pelvic floor, and the deep lumbar muscles (multifidi). Many other muscles assist in providing core stability, but this message is clear: Primary muscles of breathing, the diaphragm powering inhalation, and the TA assisting exhalation are also key to a strong and balanced core. The diaphragm is not just a breathing muscle; it helps to stabilize the rib cage when you elevate your arms and modulate intra-abdominal pressure.

Gripping the abdominal muscles in an effort to stabilize your spine activates many muscles that are not essential for core stability or breathing and may actually impede proper core control. The instruction *Pull your belly button in towards your spine* keeps the diaphragm from moving in its full range. Over time the result may be a thickened diaphragm caused by a constant shortening of its fibers. Breathing efficiently will help reach the goal of a slim waistline by teaching the diaphragm and abdominals to lengthen and shorten more fully. In yoga, dance, Pilates, or another exercise system it is important to practice the integration of breathing and stability with movement (figure 4.3). The stability function should not be given primacy to the detriment of efficient breathing. In truth, efficient breathing is a sign of biomechanically sound core control.

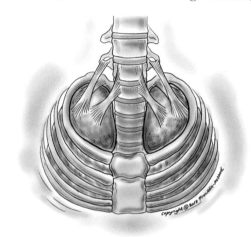

Figure 4.3 The diaphragm must be free to move, even when the core is challenged as in the Pilates leg pull.

Following are 11 exercises and imagery explorations for the breathing muscles.

Experiencing the Abdominal Muscles and Breathing

In this exercise, you will practice synchronizing breathing, stability, and movement functions of the abdominal muscles.

1. Start in a standing position. Place your fingertips below the ribs and above the pelvic crest at the side of the body. Gently push inward. Cough, laugh, or make a loud *ha* sound, and notice the strong contraction of the abdominal muscles. These muscles are helping to pull down the ribs and narrow the waistline to assist the ascent of the organs.

2. Keep your fingers in the same place, and inhale deeply. Notice that your fingers are being pushed outward. As you slowly exhale, feel how your fingers are moving inward. You are experiencing the lengthening and shortening of the abdominal wall muscle (figure 4.4). Breathing is the 24-hour conditioning of these muscles.

3. Practice gripping your abdominal muscles. As your finger test will demonstrate, the abdominal wall moves outward to a greater degree than when you fully exhale. Too much tension will not permit the abdominal muscles to slim your waistline, while exhaling will.

4. With your fingers in the same area, rotate your spine to the right and left. Laterally flex your spine to the right and left. You will feel the same muscles contracting, in this case to power movement.

5. Now, prepare to integrate movement and breathing functions. Allow the abdominal wall to move outward and inward with your breath, but at the same time perform spinal rotations and spinal lateral flexions. Notice your breathing by feeling the fingers move out and in. Allow the abdominal muscles to change simultaneously in response to breathing and your movement.

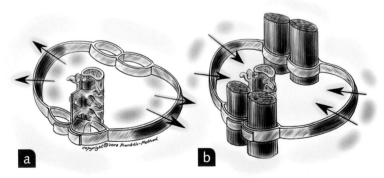

Figure 4.4   The transversus abdominis (TA) functions simultaneously in breathing to stabilize the lumbar spine and modulate the intra-abdominal pressure. *(a)* Inspiration and *(b)* expiration.

Integrating Stability, Movement, and Breathing

The following exercise can be quite challenging, especially if you have been holding your breath whenever your balance or coordination has been challenged. Practicing the following steps helps you to gain awareness of more efficient breathing concurrent with stability and movement activity.

1. Start in a standing position. Place your fingertips below the ribs and above the pelvic crest at the sides of the body. Notice how your fingers are being pushed outward during inhalation and moving inward again during exhalation.

2. Lift your right foot off the floor; you are now balancing on one leg. Did the lifting of the foot cause you to grip your breathing? Are the abdominal muscles still moving in response to breathing? Remember, the TA especially can help with stability while allowing movement for breathing.

3. To increase the challenge, you can shake the leg that is off the floor. The shaking movement will challenge the stability muscles. The TA will increase its tone as it aids the stabilizing of the lumbar spine and pelvis. However, it still needs to move in response to breathing.

4. Repeat this exercise with the other leg.

5. Perform Pilates, yoga, or dance movement or your favorite exercise with the aim of allowing unhindered breathing.

The Intercostals in Breathing and Movement Function

The intercostals comprise three layers of muscles that span the area between two ribs. Even though the function of the intercostals is not fully understood, most likely the external intercostals as well as the anterior (sternal) fibers of the internal intercostals are muscles of inspiration. The internal intercostals are muscles of forced expiration.

1. To begin, stand or sit upright. Place the tips of your thumbs between two ribs at the right and left side of your thorax. Inhale and exhale, and feel how the ribs above and below your touch lift upward and move laterally.

2. Exhale forcefully, feeling the contraction of the internal intercostals between the ribs.

3. With your thumbs remaining between two ribs on the right side, laterally flex your spine to the left. Notice how the ribs on the right are moving apart (figure 4.5). The intercostals are being stretched on the right side; on the left side, the ribs are moving together. The movement of the ribs is a result of the lateral flexion of the spine, which spreads the ribs on the contralateral side and brings them closer together on the ipsilateral side.

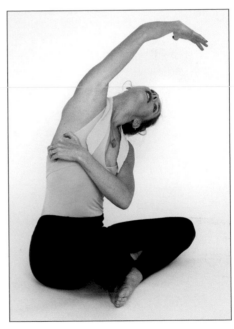

4. Laterally flex the spine to the right, and notice how the ribs on the left are spreading apart and the ribs on the right are moving together. The intercostals are being stretched on the left.

Figure 4.5 Laterally flexing your spine to the left with your fingers in the space between two ribs.

5. Now practice combining the movement function of the ribs with their breathing function. Perform lateral flexion with the goal of sensing the movement of the ribs in response to breathing as well as the movement you are performing.

(continued)

The Intercostals in Breathing and Movement Function *(continued)*

6. Move your fingers, and touch another space between two ribs. Perform lateral flexion to the right and left, and focus on the movement and breathing activity of the ribs. The goal is to be aware of both functions simultaneously.

7. Practice sensing the movement of the ribs while rotating the spine. It is more challenging to feel, but it is good practice.

8. Remove your touch, rest your arms at your sides, and take a moment to notice changes in your breathing and posture. Most likely the movement of the ribs feels easier and your spine feels taller.

How the Scalenes Support Breathing

The scalene muscles are located between the cervical spine and the upper two ribs (figure 4.6). They can lift the upper two ribs, increasing the inner thoracic volume. Without the upward pull of the scalenes, the descent of the diaphragm during inhalation would reduce the potential space for ventilating the lungs. They are therefore active whenever the diaphragm contracts. The scalene muscles also have the ability to laterally flex the neck.

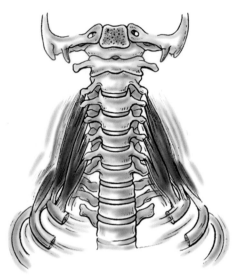

Figure 4.6   The scalene muscles.

1. Gently place your fingertips on the sides of your neck. Flex and extend your head and cervical spine. The sternocleidomastoid will be active by this movement and become prominently palpable on the side of the neck. If you feel it just in front of your fingertips, you are in the general location of the scalene muscles.

2. As you inhale, slide your fingers gently upward along the side of the neck to assist these muscles in lifting the top ribs (figure 4.7).

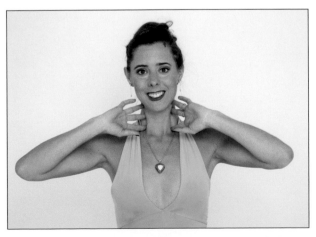

Figure 4.7   Sliding fingers up the scalenes during inhalation.

(continued)

How the Scalenes Support Breathing *(continued)*

3. As you exhale, slide your fingers downward again.

4. Repeat the upward slide during inhalation and downward slide during exhalation three times. Notice whether you can breathe more fully when assisting the scalenes with your imagery and touch.

5. To fully appreciate the correct anatomical function, it is sometimes helpful to perform the incorrect function. During inhalation slide your fingers down along the scalenes, and notice what happens to your breathing.

6. Finish the exercise by sliding your fingers upward on inhalation while also laterally flexing your neck to the right and left. The scalenes are now involved in both breath and movement.

7. Remove your touch, and notice changes. Most likely your posture is more erect and your breathing has deepened.

The Quadratus Lumborum in Breathing

The quadratus lumborum (QL) muscle attaches to the iliac crest, the first to fourth transverse processes of the lumbar spine, and the lowest rib. It can elevate the pelvis and laterally flex the spine. In breathing it serves to anchor the lowest rib to the pelvis, assisting the descent of the diaphragm.

1. Place your hands on the posterior lower rib cage. Visualize the 12th rib below your hands (figure 4.8).

2. As you inhale, slide your hands down the back toward the pelvis to support the function of the QL for breathing. Imagine the 12th rib being pulled down toward the pelvis.

3. As you exhale, slide your hands back up again.

4. Repeat the sliding and imagery three times. Notice whether the touch and imagery deepens your inhalation and lengthens your exhalation.

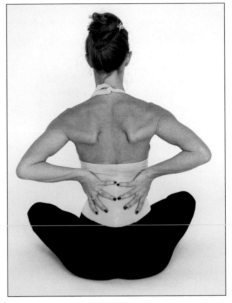

Figure 4.8 Visualizing the quadratus lumborum (QL) anchoring the 12th rib.

First and 12th Rib Movement

Creating awareness of the first and 12th ribs helps to increase the space available in your thorax for breathing. As you inhale, the first rib circle is being pulled upward by the scalenes; at the same time the 12th rib is being anchored in the opposite direction by the QL. This pull in opposite directions maximizes space in your thorax.

1. Place one hand close to your first rib circle. Place your fingers just below the clavicles where they attach to the sternum.

2. Put your other hand on the lower back in the general area of the 12th rib (figure 4.9).

3. As you inhale, imagine the first rib circle floating upward, while the 12th rib is dropping down toward the pelvis.

4. When you exhale, simply relax your mind and your touch.

5. Repeat the touch and the imagery three or four more times. Rest, noticing changes in your breathing such as a more relaxed and lengthened exhalation.

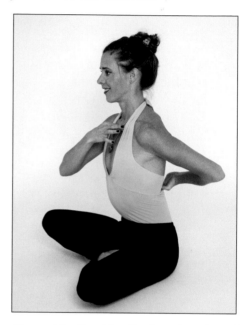

Figure 4.9 Touching the first rib circle and the 12th rib.

Ribs Coordinating With Diaphragm

The descent of the diaphragm is like a piston moving downward in its shaft. When the piston stops moving down due to the resistance of the abdominal muscles and the organs, the diaphragm assists in elevating the ribs. Both the descent of the diaphragm and the lifting of the ribs are concentric (shortening) muscle contractions of the diaphragm (figure 4.10). When you exhale the lowering of the ribs and the ascent of the diaphragm are eccentric (lengthening) actions of the diaphragm.

1. Create a model for the diaphragm and rib movement using your arms and hands. Your hands and lower arms are the dome of the diaphragm; your upper arms are the ribs.

2. Place your hands on top of each other and in front of the lower part of the sternum. Hold the elbows to the sides.

3. As you inhale, move your hands down to model the descent of the diaphragm. Mid-breath the elbows and upper arms lift to model the movement of the ribs.

4. As you exhale, perform the reverse. First the elbows and upper arms move down (the ribs), then the hands move up (the diaphragm).

5. Practice inspiration and expiration with the hand model to appreciate the coordination of diaphragm and ribs.

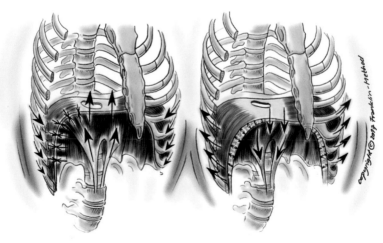

Figure 4.10   Diaphragm and rib movement.

Using a Band to Train the Muscles of Breathing

Using a band, such as a Franklin Method medium-strength band, can be an effective means to stretch and strengthen the muscles of breathing.

1. Start the exercise in a standing position with a fairly wide stance. Place the band around the middle of your back near the thoracolumbar junction. Exhaling, flex your spine while pushing into the band as if it were a hammock (figure 4.11).

2. Inhaling, return your back into extension. Use the band to push the back forward and gain more stretch.

3. Repeat this action four times, and return to the starting position.

4. Now exhaling, laterally flex your spine to the left by pushing the right side of your rib cage into the band. Your hands with the ends of the band move to the left.

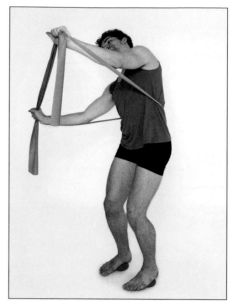

Figure 4.11 Using a band to train your breathing.

5. Returning to the starting position, inhale.

6. Exhaling, laterally flex your spine to the right by pushing the left side of your rib cage into the band. Your hands now move to the right.

7. Repeat the action four times. Remove the band, and rest. Notice any changes in your breath and posture. Most likely your rib cage feels relaxed and your posture has improved.

8. To increase the stability challenge, also perform the exercise while standing on balls. This challenge will increase the tone of the core muscles. Maintain your breathing rhythms, even now.

Stretching Your Diaphragm and Intercostals With Balls

1. Balls are helpful to stretch the muscles of breathing. In this supine exercise, use a Franklin Method water-filled mini roller to this effect. You can also use a rolled towel or two soft balls placed next to each other beneath your back.
2. Lie in the supine position and place the mini roller under your middle thoracic spine (figure 4.12).
3. Place your hands behind your head for more support.
4. Extend your spine, and lower your head to the floor.
5. Imagine and feel the stretch of the diaphragm. The sternal and crural parts of the diaphragm will be stretching especially. The anterior intercostals will be stretching as well.
6. Inhale and exhale fully to increase the stretch and toning of the diaphragm.
7. Wiggle and move your spine while breathing fully. This action stretches the fibers of the diaphragm in many directions.
8. Remove the ball and rest. Notice changes in your breathing. Your spine may feel lengthened and your shoulders more relaxed as well.

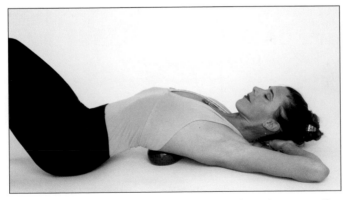

Figure 4.12   Stretching the diaphragm and intercostals with a mini roller.

Jumping With Your Breath

Not all breathing exercises need to be of the quiet nature. In this exercise you will practice the movement of the diaphragm and pelvic floor during jumping. This exercise is an example of applying your knowledge of breathing to a more challenging situation.

1. Focus on the movement of the diaphragm—down as you inhale, up when you exhale.

2. Jump up and down. Whenever you land, exhale and visualize the diaphragm rapidly moving upward (figure 4.13).

3. Inhale when you jump up.

4. Also, try the opposite: Inhale as you land, and exhale as you jump. Mostly it will feel less comfortable and more challenging. When you exhale on landing, the downward movement of the body is tempered by the upward movement of the diaphragm, allowing for a smoother and more stable landing.

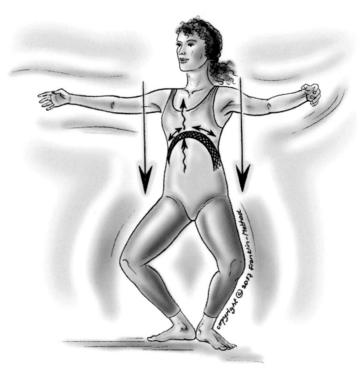

Figure 4.13 Landing from a jump with exhalation; the diaphragm moves upward.

5. Now focus also on the pelvic floor. When you land from the jump, the diaphragm moves up and the pelvic floor stretches.

6. Finally, you may add the abdominal wall to your focus. When you land and exhale, the abdominal wall will rapidly move inward, narrowing your waistline.

Daily Practice

Having a daily routine to create more optimal breathing is one of the most important activities you can do to improve your movement skills and health. Following is a selection of exercises from this book for your daily practice. However, any exercise that you have found beneficial should be added to your daily routine. Also practice breath awareness during your daily life activities, exercises, and sports.

1. *Visualizing the Diaphragm:* Visualize the movement of your diaphragm. It moves downward during inhalation and upward during exhalation. Do this visualization with hand modeling. This exercise is effective whenever you feel you need to center yourself, calm down, or make sure you are breathing efficiently. You can also combine the awareness of the diaphragm with the movement of the abdominal wall.

2. *Shaking the Diaphragm to Increase Circulation and Proprioception:* This is a fabulous way to release tension in your diaphragm and your whole body. Do not go a day without doing this exercise. Athletic teams, gymnasts, and swimmers have added this exercise to their daily routine and use it to limber up before competition.

3. *Stretching Your Diaphragm:* This is the best stretch for the muscles of breathing. Over time it will improve your breathing capacity.

4. *Tapping the Rib Cage:* Tapping the origins of the diaphragm as well as the rib cage and back helps to release tension and free your breathing for greater efficiency. You can perform this exercise with loose fists or with Franklin Method or any other soft balls.

About the Author

Eric Franklin is director and founder of the Institute for Franklin Method in Wetzikon, Switzerland. He has more than 35 years of experience as a dancer and choreographer, and he has shared imagery techniques in his teaching since 1986.

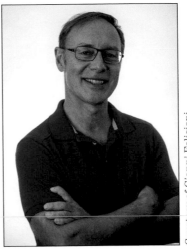

Courtesy of Gianni Felicioni

Franklin has taught extensively throughout the United States and Europe at the Juilliard School in New York, Royal Ballet School in London, Danish Ballet in Copenhagen, Dance Academy of Rome, and Institute for Psychomotor Therapy in Zurich. He was also a guest lecturer at the University of Vienna. He has provided training to Olympic and world-champion athletes and professional dance troupes such as Cirque du Soleil and the Forum de Dance in Monte Carlo. Franklin earned a BFA degree from New York University's Tisch School of the Arts and a BS degree from the University of Zurich. He has been on the faculty of the American Dance Festival since 1991.

Franklin is coauthor of the best-selling book *Breakdance*, which received a New York City Public Library Prize in 1984, and author of *100 Ideen für Beweglichkeit* and *Dance Imagery for Technique and Performance* (both books about imagery in dance and movement). He is a member of the International Association for Dance Medicine and Science.

Franklin lives near Zurich, Switzerland.

Curious to learn more?

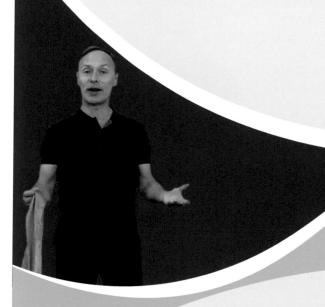